What others are saying about Improving Numeracy in Medicine

'This text is wonderfully written and clearly and concisely elucidates concepts critical for today's students, residents and practicing physicians. I'd recommend it for both undergraduate and graduate curriculum developers.'

--Saroj Misra, DO, FACOFP Director of Clinical Clerkship Curriculum for MSUCOM and Associate Program Director of Family Medicine for St. John Macomb-Oakland Hospital

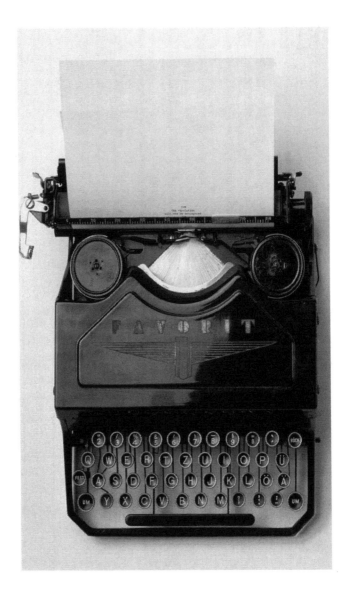

Improving Numeracy in Medicine

Published by Bonny P McClain, MSc, DC at data & donuts

Discover other titles by Bonny P McClain

Medical Writing for Smart People Because Dummies Shouldn't Write About Medicine

5 Sources for the Right Healthcare Data: Bigger Isn't Always Better

Table of Contents

A traveler's guide to the data highway

I will apologize in advance if the content of this data guidebook causes statistician's eyeballs to roll back into their sockets. It is my belief that you shouldn't need advanced study in statistics to understand the published literature. I'll be frank—research findings in medical literature are intended for the caregivers—not the statisticians. Complicated data modeling and numerical gymnastics to hopefully gain statistically significant results with barely a nod to clinical significance are problematic.

My goal is to create access by asking questions. I encourage those with advanced knowledge to join the conversation and illuminate the way for the rest of us. We need to make sense of the esoteric dialogue that surrounds data interpretation. The way patients are managed, policy is evolved, and public health questions are answered depends on it.

Many feel threatened by data analysts or others in mathematical sciences seeking qualitative understanding. One of the advances of our digital economy is the immediacy of articulating a research question and access to analytic models and tools to begin finding answers.

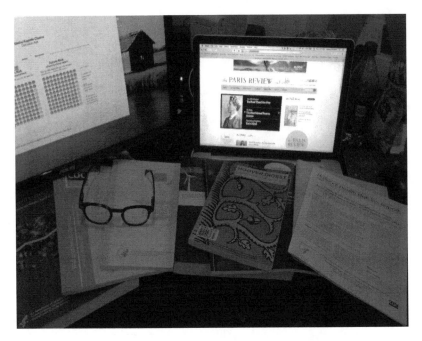

Image from my office after 2015 National Health Statistics Conference. Assimilating health data with policy implications and expert opinion informs a powerful narrative.

When I was studying as a bench scientist and analyzing microsatellite data, I had two primary questions. What was the genetic distance between the populations I was observing and what was the best mutation model? I selected several statistical software programs to help determine the frequency of the alleles in the population, the number of alleles per locus, the variance in the repeat unit, and established the presence of null alleles.

When studying population genetics, F_{st} or F-statistics measured the frequency of alleles in a population and served as a measure of genetic distance or heterozygosity. There was even software to determine the effects of demographic changes such as bottlenecks.

The objective, whether you are a scientist, clinician, journalist, or informed writer is to pursue scientific inquiry. You need to identify the role numeracy plays in our understanding of research design and interpretation. Numeracy is the ability to understand mathematical concepts and make inferences to a range of contexts and problems. For example, we can divide statistics into summaries and comparisons. Simply understanding the difference and drawbacks of either descriptive or inferential statistics can help to clarify the hypothesis or data question.

The images included are snapshots from the life of a writer—lots of travel but brief pauses to enjoy the journey.

The objective of this book isn't to make anyone an analyst or statistician but to explain what the data can and can't say—*no matter how much it is tortured* (a nod to Ronald Coase).

It seems a bit disingenuous that there is a mathematical code to be deciphered before you can be sure if the findings presented to you as fact are indeed plausible. Data is imperfect. So, the challenge is - can we create enough of an understanding to be critically vigilant when reading the literature?

Let's give it a shot.

If your experiment needs statistics, you ought to do a better experiment—Lord Ernest Rutherford

Health Literacy

We read about health literacy and targeted initiatives to improve the understanding of the complicated language reserved for discussing medicine. Now that patients are becoming shared-decision makers-- we need to foster and clarify dialogue to improve the translation of research findings, health policy, medical education, and healthcare.

I like to define health literacy as the ability to comprehend, evaluate, and negotiate data to make informed healthcare decisions or understand the peer-reviewed literature. Although we tend to think of health literacy as central to societal concerns, numeracy crosses both professional and patient populations.

For example, peer-reviewed clinical research often discusses risk-benefit analyses without the clarification that "risk" is defined as both benefits and harms. How do we calculate the harms of treatment or disease screenings to arrive at an informed clinical decision central to the patient's best interests, values, and wishes?

Statistics is the grammar of science--Karl Pearson

Numeracy

How does numeracy influence standard of care in medicine? What
does the data show us about screening healthy individuals looking for
disease upstream from illness or actual medical necessity? What do
the "results" in technical medical literature really tell us? The data is
reported in the results and abstracts of clinical literature but are we
numerate? How does the reported data extrapolate to real-world
scenarios?

I bet the majority of us have the textbooks. *Medical Statistics,
Biostatistics in Clinical Medicine, Epidemiology for Public Health Practice, The
Accidental Analyst, Essentials of Statistics,* and all of Edward Tufte's
books on data visualization are just some of the titles I can see from
my desk. But what do we know about the data in front of us? The
results of clinical research or the headlines announcing the updated
guidelines or latest findings don't necessarily translate to the point of
care? The results of our research, inevitably, must relate to what
health care providers do, or risk remaining inscrutable to and, most
likely, of minimal impact. Thus, we must answer additional questions:

How is the patient welcomed to the conversation? Shared decision-making and patient centricity requires bidirectional information exchange.

Does the media scramble the message? Often, healthcare journalists are looking to simplify and translate the results (instead of simply reporting them). We must be able to create clear, understandable outcomes to avoid the risk of misinterpretation by the public. At the end of the day, we cannot consistently blame the media or the pharmaceutical industry for this issue. They don't deliver healthcare or write prescriptions – doctors do.

Let's improve numeracy in medicine.

'Data & Donuts' is a website and blog launched to engage a motivated "tribe" in understanding the vast amount of data presented in scientific literature. In the ongoing age of evidence-based medicine, how do we draw the line between eminence-based and actual evidence?

The problem has always been the limits of numeracy in the population--especially in trying to unpack the esoteric language in clinical research. I discovered an omission of numeracy-centered education. What does a risk factor mean for the patient at the point of care? Numeracy is a language that informs. The meaning of the term is easy to gauge based on the similarity with literacy but what does it measure?

I think it is much more interesting to live with uncertainty than to live with answers that might be wrong--Richard Feynman

You will be happy to learn that complexity isn't a necessary function of numeracy. Although mathematics evolves into higher levels of difficulty, I review numeracy as the application of more fundamental skills. Numeracy begins when we strive to reason logically. The capacity to apply common patterns of mathematical thought and reason to specific logical relationships. Is a given argument logically correct?

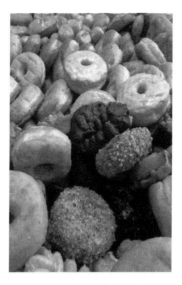

Image of donuts actually displayed on my kitchen counter. As volunteers for local efforts to feed our community we distribute donuts donated by Donut World. The Data&Donuts concept, "Come for the donuts, stay for the data," originated when trying to entice attendance at journal club meetings or an audience for research findings.

How do we critically appraise data? Understanding which are the right tools and concepts empowers us and supports the widespread agreement that mathematics is logical. Understanding how to distill logical arguments and assumptions will yield patterns of mathematical thought and reason to evidentiary review and clinical practice.

Numeracy complements literacy and is sometimes called 'mathematical literacy'. Being numerate means applying mathematical concepts in a range of contexts and communicating uncertainty in the data we collect, report, or evaluate. Being numerate is as much about thinking and reasoning logically as about 'doing maths' or 'running equations'. Rational thinking rules the day. **You can calculate the mean or average of a data set accurately but is the outcome relevant if the median was actually a better measure?**

It's not that I'm so smart; it's just that I stay with problems longer—Albert Einstein

I am a writer. I think my data journey began early when I was working on larger teams for manuscript development. The statisticians would create spreadsheets and graphics for our words. They would often write up the results sections of the manuscripts but as writers, we needed to create the narrative.

Creating health economics manuscripts requires an awareness of statistical modeling. Many health economics and outcomes research (HEOR) writers might disagree but I can't write a narrative unless I understand the framework. Why was this modeling technique utilized and not this one? How were these confidence intervals generated? Where is the non-significant data? You get the idea. The details are important when you evaluate large datasets.

Statistical software can certainly take the sting out of a meta-analysis or systematic review but you need to be aware how your upstream decisions may impact the generalizability of your findings.

Moving from general to specific, whether the research is your own or you are reviewing scientific literature—state or find the conceptual hypothesis. The next step is simply to identify the variables that will test the hypothesis. In the absence of a strong and well thought out foundation, conclusions will be of little value. At this point, either choose the appropriate statistical measures or verify that the selected models seem aligned with the research question or hypothesis.

The point of this book isn't selection of statistical tests, although once you understand your data—you will be better informed and be able to select the best options or question the adopted methodology.

At the very least, the statistics will need to answer the research question. Have the methods controlled for variables? Are the right measures elected for population comparisons?

What is the design of the study? It is important to interpret randomized, controlled, trials differently from observational studies.

The selected tests need to accommodate the limitations of design methods.

What type of data are you measuring? Are the variables numerical? Categorical? dichotomous?

As any data scientist will tell you, preparing data for analyses is typically more time consuming than the analyses. Preliminary tests should create an algorithm for how missing data is handled, outliers, multicollinearity, etc.

When analyzing data, be aware that decisions reached during the planning stages have a large impact on results — from experimental design to batch effects, lack of adjustment for confounding factors, or simple measurement error.

Important concepts

I am choosing to highlight common statistical methods. Not how we calculate statistics but what we can infer from insights derived from imperfect data samples. Uncertainty is inherent in all data samples both single populations and comparisons between populations.

The mere fact that we do not sample entire populations introduces uncertainty. We need to understand the implications of our assumptions and limitations these may create at the point of care, in creating health policy, and understanding the public health practices of our communities and society as a whole.

We must be careful not to confuse data with the abstractions we use to analyze them--William James

What data points in the literature should inform clinical decision-making? You may recall that correlation is not causation and statistical significance does not indicate clinical significance—but how are we making these determinations?

Often the well-intentioned journalist or research scientists make leaps of faith.

Abstracts are published at an alarming rate without context. Discussion of clinical significance is often trumped by statistical significance (more on that later), and homogenized clinical trial patient populations are inferred to resemble patients in a clinical practice.

If you want to test this theory go to PubMed, a "free full-text archive of biomedical and life sciences journal literature at the U.S. National Institutes of Health's National Library of medicine" and put in search terms for any medical scenario.

I am using an example from a project that I am developing—cardioprotective treatments in diabetes. The results produce 240 items, 239 with abstracts, and only 85 have free access to the entire manuscript. Is it obvious that access barriers may introduce additional levels of bias to our analyses or assumptions?

More than a few clients provide abstracts of manuscripts not freely available in PubMed or other databases. Their expectation is that abstracts are a consistently reliable source of summarized data. **This is not the case.**

The secret language of statistics, so appealing in fact-minded culture, is employed to sensationalize, inflate, confuse, and oversimplify. Statistical methods and statistical terms are necessary in reporting the mass data of social and economic trends, business conditions, "opinion" polls, the census. But without writers who use the words with honesty and understanding and readers who know what they mean, the result can only be semantic nonsense. —How to Lie with Statistics

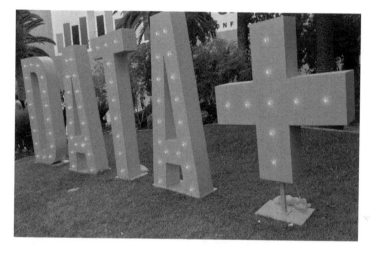

Image from Tableau Data Visualization Conference in Las Vegas.

I discuss data in a blog, Alzheimer's Disease The Brand. Much of what gets reported is generated from overzealous journalists. Here is a brief snippet that demonstrates a bit of the problem when we hobble past details when reporting. In the absence of context or the science behind the headline, the data does not support the claims.

The authors clearly refer to Aβ transmission and not transmission of Alzheimer's disease, as none of the patients had clinical AD or the tangles that in addition to Aβ deposits are required to make a postmortem diagnosis of AD.

Is Alzheimer's Disease Transmissible? | Medpage Today
www.medpagetoday.com/.../AlzheimersDisease/53458 ▾ MedPage Today ▾
Sep 9, 2015 - In rare circumstances, Alzheimer's disease might be transmissible, a study suggested. "In addition to sporadic Alzheimer's disease and ...

Could Alzheimer's Disease Be Transmissible? - Newsweek
www.newsweek.com/could-alzheimers-disease-be-transmissible-371247 ▾
Sep 11, 2015 - A new study suggests that the 'seeds' of Alzheimer's disease could be spread from person to person.

Alzheimer's Disease May Be Transmissible, Study Finds
www.livescience.com/18406-alzheimers-disease-transmission-prion-mad... ▾
Oct 5, 2011 - In some cases, Alzheimer's disease may in fact be the result of an infection, and may be even be transmissible, a new study in mice suggests. In the study, mice injected with human brain tissue from Alzheimer's patients developed Alzheimer's disease.

Is the Alzheimer's protein contagious? | Science/AAAS | News
news.sciencemag.org/brain.../2015/.../alzheimer-s-protein-contagiou... ▾ Science ▾
Sep 9, 2015 - Still unknown in Alzheimer's is what role misfolded proteins such as amyloid-β and tau play in the disease, and whether they are transmissible through direct contact with or consumption of contaminated brain tissue.

No, Alzheimer's is not contagious - CNN.com
www.cnn.com/2015/09/10/health/no-alzheimers-is-not-contagious ▾ CNN ▾
Sep 10, 2015 - "Alzheimer's disease may be infectious," The Independent wrote ... that Alzheimer's disease is transmissible, notably by blood transfusions.

Autopsies reveal signs of Alzheimer's in growth-hormone ...
www.nature.com/.../autopsies-reveal-signs-of-alzheimer-s-in-growth-... ▾ Nature ▾
Sep 9, 2015 - Only a decade ago, the idea that Alzheimer's disease might be transmissible between people would have been laughed off the stage.

Alzheimer's disease may be infectious, study claims - Health
www.independent.co.uk › ... › Health News ▾ The Independent ▾
Sep 10, 2015 - The investigation has shown for the first time in humans that Alzheimer's disease may be a transmissible infection which could be inadvertently ...

Alzheimer's Disease | Deadly. Transmissible. Unstoppable.

You can see how the article created a bit of a news bump and hysteria in some less medical or scientifically inclined news agencies.

There is no way to determine if these people would have developed Alzheimer's disease. The protein was observed in seven of the eight brains examined.

The findings are fascinating but the sample size is way too small to draw any conclusions.

Other hallmarks of Alzheimer's disease, such as tau protein, were not discovered in any cases. Beta-amyloid protein deposits occur in the brain as a part of aging and are not an indicative precursor for dementia or Alzheimer's disease.

A few other consistent errors to look out for...

My biggest "pebble in shoe" aggravation stems from:

- Use of odds and probability interchangeably,

- Reporting relative risks without consideration of absolute risk calculations,

- Confusing correlation with causation

- Not paying appropriate attention to whether findings are in animal or human models, or in a large enough population to detect a difference (if one exists).

Lets briefly introduce the difference between odds and probability here. I typically revert to coin flips to help clarify the difference. Both odds and probability describe the chance of an event occurring. The odds describe the estimated probability of the event occurring, divided by the estimated probability of it not occurring.

Back to the coin flip. The odds of getting tails are 1:1. You either get heads or you get tails. Now probability is slightly different. You can either get heads or tails (numerator) but there is the probability of two events (heads and tails) in the denominator. The probability is now 50%.

If you want to think about this medically, let's think of a scenario where we give a drug to 10 patients (small for illustrative purposes). Unfortunately, 6 of the patients have a stroke. The probability of having a stroke is 6/10 or 0.6. So what are the odds? 6/4? The odds are 1.5. The difference is all in the denominator—for probability it is "all the cases" and we have a maximum value of 1. For odds we are interested in the patients that did not have a stroke and the values are infinite.

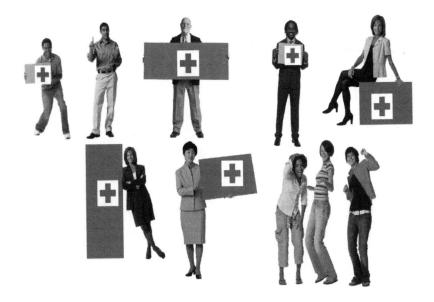

In summary, because a probability is a number between 0 and 1, the probability of having a stroke is 60%. Now if we are looking at odds we are saying that for every 10 patients, 6 of them will have a stroke, and 4 of them will not.

Here is my simple comment about correlation not being the same as causation. Today I had whole grain toast with fresh avocado for breakfast. And then I headed to the pool. A great workout if I say so myself. As a triathlete, the swim is always tough and I spend a lot of time refining skills and striving to improve. Today the laps seemed almost effortless; I kept the stroke count down (a sign of efficiency) and emerged from the pool feeling victorious.

Wow. Who knew that toast with avocado could improve my swim times AND efficiency? You see where I am going here? There are a lot of other independent variables at play that may have a stronger link to my results. How many hours did I sleep on average the night before? Did I skip my long run the day before? What was the temperature of the pool? Did I wear my lucky swim cap? Take home message here is to encourage awareness of the influence of multiple independent variables when stating summary statements or conclusions.

We are able to infer correlation but without experimental or interventional assessments we are unable to infer causation. Speaking from a clinical standpoint--observational studies (assessing correlation) in the real world but in the absence of experimentation are cited in the media more than experimental or randomized controlled trials (RCTs), which are more reliable.

Observational studies look at large populations but the weakness is that all variables are not controlled and as you know, the unknown variables confound such studies.

When reading research findings you should be able to determine the following:

- Multiple literature reviews support these ideas and many variations of a similar theme.
- How was the study designed?
- Was the research question stated clearly?
- Is the study population aligned with clinical need?
- Are the methods appropriate?
- Do the authors describe how the data was collected?
- Are the analyses described with enough detail that they could be replicated?
- Is the research presented clearly using appropriate tables and graphics that clarify, not distort the findings?
- How big are the findings?
- What are the harms, adverse events, costs?
- Could the finding be wrong?
- Interpretation should discuss limitations of research design and what additional data questions remain—are the conclusions substantive?
- Are financial disclosures and/or study sponsors mentioned?

Clinical Trials

There are many resources for exhaustive discussions about research design. I tend to rely on the International Society for Pharmacoeconomics and Outcomes Research (ISPOR) or Institute for Clinical and Economic Review (ICER). My intention is to provide an overview for context when we discuss data from the literature. The biggest take-away should be an understanding of how to evaluate the uncertainty in estimates provided by different types of research design and evaluation.

Before we look at data—we have to collect it. Let's start with the clinical trial. You may have heard of the Consolidated Standards of Reporting Trials Statement (CONSORT) and tools to address inadequate reporting of randomized controlled trials. Data quality and interpretation should be approached with an arched eyebrow. Clinical trial data can be a marketer's dream. How endpoints, comparators, trial length, and other variables are selected can directly influence the outcomes and distort findings to support brand messages or clearly communicate research findings (hopefully). How do you determine the difference?

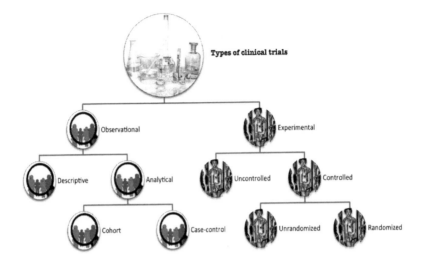

Types of clinical trials

Observational — Descriptive, Analytical (Cohort, Case-control)

Experimental — Uncontrolled, Controlled (Unrandomized, Randomized)

"You can't fix by analysis what you bungled by design." --Light, Singer and Willett

The gold standard is the randomized controlled trial or RCT. These trials are randomly allocated interventional studies where exposure to a specific device or treatment is controlled between different groups. Ideally RCTs are double-blinded and neither the patients nor investigators are aware of group assignment. We are then able to measure the size of the difference in a pre-defined set of clinical endpoints or outcomes. The characteristics of a sample should (imperfectly) mirror those of the larger population; we can only estimate findings applicable to the overall population.

Meta-analyses combine results from multiple studies to reach a single conclusion with greater statistical power than the individual studies alone. Systematic reviews and meta-analyses have the ability to summarize a large body of evidence and explain variability of individual study findings and help contextualize the need for new studies or data.

The only systematic difference between randomized groups in clinical trials should be the exposure of interest, i.e., assigned therapy or intervention. The RCTs are the top of the hierarchy because we can make important assumptions for our analyses based on our data. We can assume that because the sample population is random we can generalize findings to the population. Randomization tends to ensure that any confounding variables that exist will be evenly distributed among the treatment arms or active and control populations.

Nonrandomized studies are also able to detect associations but we are unable to determine if the association was caused by another factor such as a relationship between two of the independent variables. Unrecognized confounders can distort the potential differences between treatment groups and placebo or alternative treatment options.

No matter the clinical trial design, the benefit should be weighed against any harms or costs.

Cohort studies start with the exposure. The exposure is typically a specific therapy. Some individuals have been exposed to a treatment and some have not—and then we look for the outcome of interest over time. The outcome can be a heart attack or other clinical endpoint. Statistically we can calculate the risk of heart attack in patients exposed to the treatment in question and those patients not exposed to the treatment.

In a **case-control study** you actually start with an outcome. Perhaps you are looking at patients with a certain outcome, some cases have the outcome others don't. We work backwards and look for exposure. In rare diseases--odds and probability are almost the same. This makes sense if you recall that case control studies are most commonly used for rare diseases.

Non-interventional clinical studies are often retrospective. Although they include comparisons between treatment groups, they are not randomized but provided therapy at the clinician's discretion and typically in consideration of a patient's preferences. If you keep in mind the "direction" of the data collection you can easily keep the two concepts clear. In a simplified prospective study you begin with a sample of healthy subjects that are either exposed or not exposed to a particular risk or intervention. We can then measure if they develop the endpoint or illness. Retrospective we actually look for the exposure, examine illness, and make assumptions about the population.

A standard metric or heuristic to apply when interpreting reported data should include information about the design of the study, clearly articulated research question (hypothesis), proper selection of statistical models (should be clearly stated in methods), interpretation of results and the appropriateness of substantive conclusions.

Clinical trial data typically examines an active arm and a comparator or control group. How do we measure benefit of an investigative drug over the control (either a placebo or another standard of care)? We can look to the relative risk, the relative risk reduction, or the odds ratio. For clinical decision-making, however, it is more clinically meaningful to use the measure "number needed to treat (NNT)" – more on NNT later.

What type of data do you have?

There are statistical methods appropriate for different types of data. I am not recommending specific algorithms but you can find information for the type of analyses, software program, and data type—there really isn't a "one size fits all" approach so stay vigilant.

You might be familiar with continuous data, binary data, categorical data, and time to event data (survival data).

The most important thing to recall from continuous data is that one incremental change in value is the same across the full range of data values. For example, a change in blood pressure, age, or weight has a comparative value.

Binary data is also called dichotomous data and as the name suggests it is either "yes" or "no". If you have more than one category, your data is now classified as categorical. If you were to blend binary and continuous data you would have time to event data. Does the event occur? And what was the time to event (occurrence) or event –free time point.

- Categorical or qualitative data includes:
  - Binary: two choices
    - Yes or no
    - Dead or alive
    - Disease-free or disease
- Nominal: more than two choices (no order)
  - Race
  - Age group
- Ordinal: more than two choices but ordered or ranked
  - Stages of cancer
  - Likert scales

Difference in the means

Recall that the measurement of any sample of data is imperfect. If your data sample is small the mean or sample average is likely not close to the true mean of the population. The benefit of a larger sample size is the increased precision of estimates of the population level. Descriptive statistical calculations combine measures of central tendency (mean, median, mode) and variability (standard deviation or interquartile range) to generate a confidence interval (CI) for the population mean.

Normal Distribution

The central limit theorem says that if samples are large enough, the distribution of means will follow a normal distribution even if the population is not "normal".

Since most statistical tests (such as the t test and ANOVA) are concerned only about differences between means, the Central Limit Theorem lets these tests work well even when the populations are not normal. The catch is that the samples have to be reasonably large. How large is that? It depends on how far the population distribution differs from a normal distribution.

Biological data never strictly follow a normal distribution precisely, because a normal distribution extends infinitely in both directions, including both infinitely low negative numbers and infinitely high positive numbers in the tails of the curve. **But many kinds of biological data follow a bell-shaped distribution that is approximately normal.**

An alternative statistical approach does not assume that data follow a normal distribution. These tests are called nonparametric tests but as you may have guessed, they are less powerful than parametric tests that assume normal distributions.

The normal distribution assumes the '68-95-99.7' rule. A total of 68% of the observations are within one standard deviation of the mean, 95% are within two standard deviations and 99.7 are within 3 standard deviations.

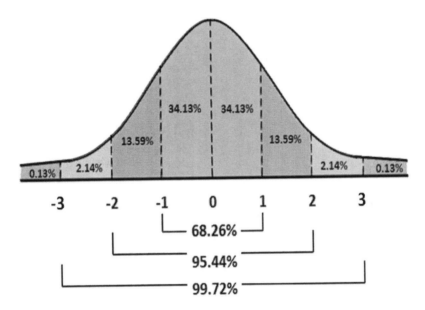

You can calculate intervals for any desired degree of confidence, but 95% confidence intervals are used most commonly in the scientific literature. If you assume that your sample is randomly selected (normal) you are 95% sure that the confidence interval includes the population mean. More precisely, if you generate many 95% CIs from many data sets, you expect the CI to include the true population mean in 95% of the cases and not to include the true mean value in the other 5%. It is impossible to know the true population mean, but you can estimate.

So how do we discuss uncertainty in our estimates?

Assume that you've collected data from two samples, and the means are different. You want to know whether the data were sampled from populations with different means. Observing different sample means is not enough to persuade you to conclude that the populations are different. It is possible that the populations have the same mean, and the difference you observed is a coincidence of random sampling.

There is no way you can ever be sure whether the difference you observed reflects a true difference or a coincidence of random sampling. All you can do is calculate the probabilities. Inferential statistics are used to make generalizations from a sample to a population using the theory of probabilities. Slightly better than relying on divine intervention.

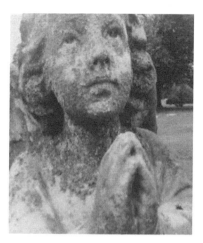

P-value

I can't tell you how many of us have been in a twist about understanding the null hypothesis (myself included). Think about it like this. We are going to assume that there will be no difference between our comparator groups. The active arm and control arm or the comparator therapy—no difference. You will fail to reject the hypothesis unless you see enough evidence to reject. This is your null hypothesis—there is no difference between groups.

In medical research it has been decided that the maximum p-value where we will reject the null hypothesis is alpha (significance level) and is 0.05. When the p-value is less than alpha we call the hypothesis test statistically significant. There are other levels but we will only discuss the industry standard in the medical literature.

There is always the chance that you have a type 1 error, incorrectly rejecting the null hypothesis. The P-value is the probability that a type 1 error was made. If researchers find a difference between two treatment arms for example, they don't want it to be due to chance. In scientific research we typically preset the threshold for the p-value. **When the P-value < alpha, reject the null. When P-value > alpha, fail to reject the null.**

A hypothesis test tells us whether the observed data are consistent with the null hypothesis, and a confidence interval tells us which hypotheses are consistent with the data--William C. Blackwelder

The P value is a probability, with a value ranging from zero to one. If the P value is small (typically < .05), you'll conclude that the difference is quite unlikely to be caused by random sampling. You'll conclude instead that the populations have different means for example.

Misinterpretation of P value

There are many misinterpretations of p-values but one of the main mistakes is made when confusing statistical significance with clinical significance. The p-value doesn't tell you anything about the rigor of the research question. This is why p-values by themselves don't tell us anything. A best practice is to always report p-values with confidence intervals. A large enough sample size can detect a small difference between populations (when one really may not exist) revealing a Type I error—probability of failing to reject the null hypothesis when you should.

It is important to note that statistical significance only rules out random sampling as the cause of the findings. Not rejecting the null hypothesis is not the same as accepting the null as true. We either reject the null hypothesis or fail to reject the null hypothesis. There are different alpha levels for p-values but the research standard is 0.05.

Also be concerned if you read phrases like "approaching significance" or "trending toward significance," they mean absolutely nothing.

More about the null hypothesis

Because we are making assumptions from imperfect data we focus on testing the null hypothesis. Are the findings the result of chance? **The p-value can tell us if what we see in the data occurred by chance alone.** Intuitively you may conclude that the probability of the null hypothesis being correct decreases with larger sample sizes. This can be an interesting artifact. The .05 value is arbitrary. Should we take note of small differences between groups that get statistically significant with a larger sample of the population?

This is where the effect-size becomes necessary. We need a measure to determine the sizes of associations. The most common in the scientific literature are correlation/regression coefficients r and R. Correlation is how different variables relate to one another.

Correlation coefficient r describes the range of "0" or no relationship whatsoever to a perfect relationship "1, or -1", independently of sample size. The negative or positive just shows if it is a positive or negative association. When interpreting effect sizes, an r of ".1" represents a 'small' effect size, ".3" represents a 'medium' effect size and ".5" represents a 'large' effect size. I am reporting industry standards from memory and will include a list of resources and recommended reading to support the practices at the end of the book.

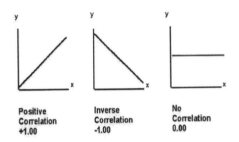

Positive
Correlation
+1.00

Inverse
Correlation
-1.00

No
Correlation
0.00

The correlation coefficient measures the strength of linear relationship between two variables and is bounded between -1 and 1, inclusive.

Correlations close to zero represent no linear association between the variables, whereas correlations close to -1 or +1 indicate strong linear relationship. Intuitively, the easier it is for you to draw a line of best fit through a scatterplot, the more correlated they are. The regression slope measures the "steepness" of the linear relationship between two variables and can take any value from $-\infty$ to $+\infty$.

Slopes near zero mean that the response (Y) variable changes slowly as the predictor (X) variable changes. Slopes that are further from zero (either in the negative or positive direction) mean the response changes more rapidly as the predictor changes. Intuitively, if you were to draw a line of best fit through a scatterplot, the steeper it is, the further your slope is from zero.

Correlation is not causation, but it sure is a hint—Edward Tufte

So the correlation coefficient and regression slope MUST have the same sign (+ or -), but will almost never have the same value

Cohen's d is another measure of effect size. When comparing two means, Cohen's d is the difference in the two groups' means divided by the average of their standard deviations. This means that if we see a d of 1, we know that the two groups' means differ by one standard deviation; a d of .5 tells us that the two groups' means differ by half a standard deviation; and so on. Cohen suggested that d=0.2 be considered a 'small' effect size, 0.5 represents a 'medium' effect size and 0.8 a 'large' effect size.

This means that if two groups' means don't differ by 0.2 standard deviations or more, the difference is trivial, even if it is statistically significant. Although you often see Cohen's D values published I would argue that they aren't intuitive clinically. The number needed to treat (NNT), on the other hand relates effect size directly to the point of care—more on that later.

Confidence intervals

If you recall, the Central Limit Theorem states that all random samples generated from a population of a size "n", should have summary statistics computed (mean, proportion, incidence rate) with the distribution of those values (95%) falling within 2 standard deviations of the true value they are estimating. **The CI provides a range of uncertainty.**

This 95% confidence interval is the typical industry standard—a range of possible values based on different levels of uncertainty. It means that 95% of the randomly selected samples will contain the true or actual measure of interest.

As you might imagine, there are a few assumptions. Typically the sample size cut-off is n=60. Or at least that was the case back when the majority of these calculations were done by hand. Now in a modern age of computer simulations, CI can be calculated for any sample size. What happens when n< 60?

This is when we say the sampling distribution follows a t-distribution. Because there is more variability in a smaller sample, calculations extend beyond the 2 standard errors or deviations to reach 95% under the sampling distribution. There are tables that will compute degrees of freedom.

No need to worry. We still interpret the 95% CI the same regardless of how it was computed. Confidence interval limits are comparable on the log scale similarly to ratios as discussed before. The most important thing to remember is to be sure that your CI does not cross the value of no effect—"1" for ratios or "0" for differences.

Power

You may have assumed (correctly) that because there is a Type 1
error, there must be a Type 2 error. Well here it is. Assume you did
not observe a statistically significant difference between two
treatments. What percent of time would we accept the null
hypothesis if the null hypothesis should actually be rejected?

You fail to reject the null hypothesis. Are you sure? Did the study
have the power to detect differences? Power is the probability of
finding a difference between the groups if two groups are different.
This is most important in negative studies. The main determinant is
sample size. A type II error, instead of alpha, we think of beta.

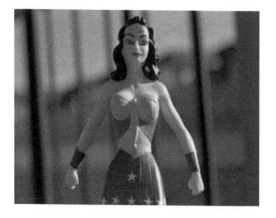

Researchers typically determine that the threshold of power will be at
least 80%. Power calculations will determine power of study design.

Power = 1 –beta. Increased sample size, effect size, and precision increase power (standard deviation decreasing). Researchers don't arbitrarily decide on the "n" of a study. They recruit for the level of power they hope to have in their study.

Rule of thumb

Report absolute risks for each group. When considering risk, be certain you know the outcome measure (heart attack, mortality, survival?), what time period the outcome occurred (time interval, e.g., 3 years), and in what population (adults with a specific diagnosis).

Without data you're just another person with an opinion—
W.Edwards Deming

The number needed to treat (NNT)

The clinician needs an intuitive tool or statistic to compare benefits and risks of prevention, diagnosis, and alternate therapeutic approaches.

Why not just use the relative risk and odds ratios? What I observed from looking at many datasets is that the RR seems to depend more on what happens in the control or standard care arm. For example if you assume a 25% benefit with treatment but vary the incidence in the control group the RR can fluctuate quite a bit even with a constant 30% benefit.

The NNT is a statistical construct to help balance benefits with harms or at least the effect size of a given intervention. Some patients will receive benefit, others are harmed, and some are not affected at all. Knowing the NNT won't really tell you anything about the patient in front of you but at least it scales to the patient level. The ideal number needed to treat is 1, indicating that all treated patients will benefit. Less effective treatments have higher values. It becomes even more complex when looking at benefit in treatment vs. preventative strategies. Keep this in mind when observing NNTs greater than 10 or more.

This measure is calculated on the inverse of the absolute risk reduction. It has the advantage that it conveys both statistical and clinical significance to the doctor. Furthermore, it can be used to extrapolate published findings to a patient at an arbitrary specified baseline risk when the relative risk reduction associated with treatment is constant for all levels of risk. You can ignore the sign of the NNT as long as you understand the difference when looking at a treatment NNT vs. a preventative or diagnostic NNT. Let's unpack some of these terms and then look at the literature to see how a new understanding may lead to new insights.

Limitations of NNT

You may have noticed NNT being included beyond just descriptions of individualized benefits or even harms. The application of NNT to cost benefit analyses and the introduction of confidence intervals and questions of validity are often beyond the average observer.

It suffices to be aware that there is a lack of consensus of preferred methods for calculating NNT confidence intervals because they produce different results. In the meanwhile most studies you see will be difference between means with their associated confidence intervals and significance testing.

Not necessarily a limitation if addressed adequately but when comparing multiple clinical trials in a meta-analysis for example, NNTs are time dependent. The follow-up years need to be converted although changes in benefit and harm are not consistent.

Number needed to harm

Calculating harms is identical to NNT but we are now describing adverse events. For example, large numbers are actually good for NNH as they indicate that adverse events are rare. Be mindful that when clinical trials are stopped early due to benefit of active arm, this can distort the data. We anticipate that more adverse events will accumulate over time so when a clinical trial is stopped prematurely we lose much needed long-term data.

Many research articles list the serious adverse events in a table. You can report them just like NNT with a little nudge to the language. For example, If the NNH is 100, "For every 100 people treated with drug x compared to drug y, there will be one more case of syncope"… it is important to create context around the harm associated with the treatment. The higher the NNH the better, meaning that the more patients that are seen without the event, the more benefit associated with the treatment.

It can be useful to calculate "likelihood to be helped or harmed" or LHH, the ratio of NNH to NNT. The ratio greater than 1 would be desired when comparing a positive outcome or less than or equal to 1 if comparing a desired outcome with an adverse event that is usually mild or moderate, usually temporary and does not lead to discontinuation, or there is a particularly urgent need for benefit (efficacy) that mitigates an otherwise prohibitive risk of harm (side effects).

Number needed to screen

The number needed to screen (NNS) is the reciprocal of the absolute difference in cumulative mortality. To calculate NNS, we need to know the background risk, or prevalence, of the particular disease to be detected in the population to be screened, and the mortality rate of the disease in patients screened and not screened.

These statistics are time specific and will change as the risks for the treatment groups either converge or diverge over time. Values for number needed to treat (NNT) and number needed to screen (NNS) reported at single time points may distort time to event data as mortality differences diverge at longer time intervals--decreasing NNT projections.

Hazard Ratio

What is a hazard ratio? An important differentiation between relative risk and hazard ratio is that the hazard ratio is the averaged measure of risk over the entire study period. Time to event analysis is basically the time for an event to occur. In contrast to a relative risk we aren't worried about timing of events, just total number of events. We view the two dimensions in a survival curve, typically the Kaplan-Meier method. These provide graphic detail to incidence rate ratios.

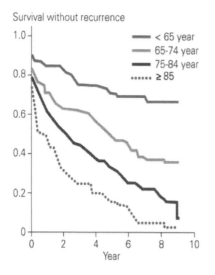

The term "hazard" used in this context might seem strange but it is referring to the probability that an individual at time "t" has an event at that time—it's an instantaneous event rate. Because the HR is a ratio, a HR of 1 means the number of events is the same in both arms. As people accrued events they are plotted on the graph. Recall that as time interval increases we anticipate seeing fewer people recorded as event free.

Odds Ratio

A third summary measure, the odds ratio answers the question, what is the relative likelihood of a certain outcome. It differs from relative risk reduction (RRR) because it isn't comparing ratio of probabilities of different adverse outcomes, it is the ratio of the odds of adverse outcomes. Think of it as the estimated probability of an event, divided by the estimated probability that it won't occur. As the numerator or "risk" increases, so do the odds.

The OR is often used as a valid measure of treatment effect in RCT but it also can be insensitive to differences in magnitude of risk without therapy. What is the ratio in favor of a certain outcome for the treatment group compared to the odds in favor of the same outcome in the control group? It is helpful to remember that if the outcome is common (AR >20%), odds ratios often overstate the effects. Always report ARs in each exposure group as well.

The range of possible values for positive and negative associations is different. The ratio-based associations are differ in magnitude as the direction of comparison is reversed. When the association is negative (reduced risk in numerator) the range of possible values lies between 0 and 1.

When the association is positive (increased risk in numerator) the range of possible values lies between 1 and infinity. Scale of ratios is not symmetric. The ranges are equal though, on the ln (ratio) scale.

The bigger the number, the more impressive. When should you believe? Compare unadjusted RR or OR to one variable with at least 1 known confounder adjusted. If the adjustment produces a large decline in the OR or the RR be suspicious of a spurious association. In contrast if the adjustment increases the RR or OR or if it remains stable then we can be more confident in the validity of the association.

Unadjusted RR = no of cases in exposure group/number of total in group divided by no of cases in non-exposed group/number in total group. Compare this to the adjusted. Many times both adjusted and unadjusted values are provided. It is worthwhile to do a few calculations even if they haven't been presented in the research findings.

Regression Analysis 101

Regression analysis is a method to test the relationship and significance between dependent variable (y-axis) and independent variable (x-axis). In research, independent variables (age, religion, married, gender) might be important determinants to measure against the dependent variable. How do we know if they correlate?

We try to understand what happens to the dependent variable if the independent variable changes. You take observations and try to find a line that fits through all of the points—a regression line based on least squares method.

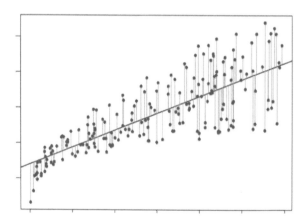

What is the difference between the actual values and estimated values? Is the number positive or negative? It will be easier to describe when looking at actual data so for now we are looking at the strength of relationships. Estimates indicate the slope of a line that would be drawn to connect the various values.

Research can be complex when we are looking to predict the value of a variable. Often we can get better predictions if we use more than one variable. In multiple regression, the dependent variable is predicted by two or more variables.

Briefly, multiple regression is an extension of simple linear regression (SLR). Recall that SLR is a one to one relationship. We are exploring the relationship between an independent variable and a dependent variable to make predictions. Many think that multiple independent variables make the regression better but it is equally likely that over-fitting may occur.

It is true that variation can be explained better with more independent variables but it can also open a Pandora's box.

Pick the best variables for the model.

The addition of more independent variables creates more relationships among them. This additional set of independent variables may not only be related to the dependent variable but may potentially be related to each other. This is called multicollinearity. **The ideal is for independent variables to be correlated with the dependent variable but not each other.**

Example from the literature...

Systolic Blood Pressure Intervention Trial (SPRINT)

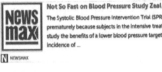

Not So Fast on Blood Pressure Study Zeal

The Systolic Blood Pressure Intervention Trial (SPRINT) trial was stopped prematurely because subjects in the intensive treatment group (the aim was to study the benefits of a lower blood pressure target) had a significantly lower incidence of ...

N NEWSMAX

More Intensive Blood Pressure Management Can Save Lives, SPRINT Study Finds

This was the finding of a landmark clinical trial sponsored by the National Institutes of Health (NIH) called the Systolic Blood Pressure Intervention Trial (SPRINT), published online today in the New England Journal of Medicine, and being presented at ...

F FORBES

SPRINT study: Aim for lower blood pressure target to save lives

The Systolic Blood Pressure Intervention Trial (SPRINT), which enrolled more than 9,300 individuals who were older than 50 and had at least one other risk factor for heart disease, was ended a year early because of its lifesaving information, the ...

DRUG TOPICS

The media was quick to report the efficacy of lowering blood pressure targets in the absence of data.

This is a quick snapshot of a variety of stories heralding the study as a landmark on one end of the spectrum and debunking its value on the other.

Lets review some of the data and content to see the merit in the research findings or which patients (if any) may benefit from intensive blood pressure lowering.

The point isn't to discredit any of the reported research findings. The goal is to create awareness around data and reveal insights that might be hidden below the surface. I found this clinical trial of particular interest because the headlines were mostly sensationalized without any of the data available at the time most headlines went to press.

Considerations when reviewing literature:

- How was the study designed?

- Was the research question stated clearly?

- Is the primary outcome a surrogate? Does it strongly link to patient outcomes?

- If a composite endpoint, what do you know about the role of each component?

- Is the study population aligned with clinical need?

- Are the methods appropriate?

- Do the authors describe how the data was collected?

- How big is the result? What are the harms? Could it be wrong?

- Are the analyses described with enough detail that they could be replicated?

- Is the research presented clearly using appropriate tables and graphics that clarify, not distort the findings?

- Interpretation should discuss limitations of research design and what additional data questions remain—are the conclusions substantive?

- Are financial disclosures and/or study sponsors mentioned?

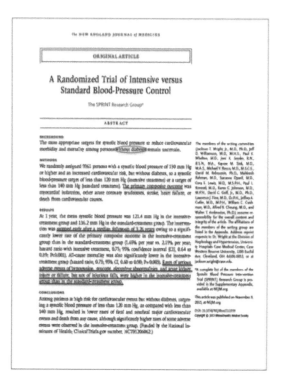

How was the study designed?

Although the study was randomized and controlled, it is open-label. This means that patients and investigators are aware of treatment assignment—this can potentially introduce bias.

Was the research question stated clearly?

Is the study population aligned with clinical need? The population is excluding patients with diabetes—a usual representative at-risk demographic.

Are the methods appropriate?

When I see composite outcomes I am reminded of stacking the deck—trying to increase the likelihood of reaching statistical significance. Often composite outcomes in time to event trials lead to higher event rates and enable smaller sample sizes or shorter follow-up (often both). A substantive risk associated with the reporting of composite outcomes is that the benefits described may be presumed to relate to all of the components.

The authors report NNT to prevent a primary outcome event (first occurrence of myocardial infarction, acute coronary syndrome, stroke, heart failure, or death from cardiovascular causes) death from any cause, and death from cardiovascular causes.

None of the values are compelling and I might argue they are in fact confusing. For example, the NNT to prevent a primary outcome event during the median 3.26 years of the trial was 61 (I calculated 63 but rounding differences may account for fluctuations). This means that for every 63 patients on intensive treatment one primary outcome event would be prevented.

But which primary outcome? There are 4 listed in the outcome. And now with cardiovascular causes also listed as a separate NNT we see that **for every 172 patients treated with intensive treatment one death from cardiovascular cause is prevented.**

The rate of the primary composite outcome was 1.65 percent per year in the intensive group and 2.19 percent per year in the standard group, a difference of .54 percent although the press release reported the relative risk reduction. Death from any cause occurred in 155 adults in the intensive group and 210 adults in the standard group, a 27% reduction for intensive treatment compared to standard.

Table 2. Primary and Secondary Outcomes and Renal Outcomes.*

Outcome	Intensive Treatment		Standard Treatment		Hazard Ratio (95% CI)	P Value
	no. of patients (%)	% per year	no. of patients (%)	% per year		
All participants	**(N= 4678)**		**(N= 4683)**			
Primary outcome†	243 (5.2)	1.65	319 (6.8)	2.19	0.75 (0.64–0.89)	<0.001
Secondary outcomes						
Myocardial infarction	97 (2.1)	0.65	116 (2.5)	0.78	0.83 (0.64–1.09)	0.19
Acute coronary syndrome	40 (0.9)	0.27	40 (0.9)	0.27	1.00 (0.64–1.55)	0.99
Stroke	62 (1.3)	0.41	70 (1.5)	0.47	0.89 (0.63–1.25)	0.50
Heart failure	62 (1.3)	0.41	100 (2.1)	0.67	0.62 (0.45–0.84)	0.002
Death from cardiovascular causes	37 (0.8)	0.25	65 (1.4)	0.43	0.57 (0.38–0.85)	0.005
Death from any cause	155 (3.3)	1.03	210 (4.5)	1.40	0.73 (0.60–0.90)	0.003
Primary outcome or death	332 (7.1)	2.25	423 (9.0)	2.90	0.78 (0.67–0.90)	<0.001
Participants with CKD at baseline	**(N= 1330)**		**(N= 1316)**			
Composite renal outcome‡	14 (1.1)	0.33	15 (1.1)	0.36	0.89 (0.42–1.87)	0.76
≥50% reduction in estimated GFR§	10 (0.8)	0.23	11 (0.8)	0.26	0.87 (0.36–2.07)	0.75
Long-term dialysis	6 (0.5)	0.14	10 (0.8)	0.24	0.57 (0.19–1.54)	0.27
Kidney transplantation	0		0			
Incident albuminuria¶	49/526 (9.3)	3.02	59/500 (11.8)	3.90	0.72 (0.48–1.07)	0.11
Participants without CKD at baseline	**(N= 3332)**		**(N= 3345)**			
≥30% reduction in estimated GFR to <60 ml/min/1.73 m²§	127 (3.8)	1.21	37 (1.1)	0.35	3.49 (2.44–5.10)	<0.001
Incident albuminuria¶	110/1769 (6.2)	2.00	135/1831 (7.4)	2.41	0.81 (0.63–1.04)	0.10

* CI denotes confidence interval, and CKD chronic kidney disease.
† The primary outcome was the first occurrence of myocardial infarction, acute coronary syndrome, stroke, heart failure, or death from cardiovascular causes.
‡ The composite renal outcome for participants with CKD at baseline was the first occurrence of a reduction in the estimated GFR of 50% or more, long-term dialysis, or kidney transplantation.
§ Reductions in the estimated GFR were confirmed by a second laboratory test at least 90 days later.
¶ Incident albuminuria was defined by a doubling of the ratio of urinary albumin (in milligrams) to creatinine (in grams) from less than 10 at baseline to greater than 10 during follow-up. The denominators for number of patients represent those without albuminuria at baseline.
‖ No long-term dialysis or kidney transplantation was reported among participants without CKD at baseline.

Now that you are aware of NNH, there is data provided that allows calculations. For example if you look at the risk of hypotension (remember to look at p-values and confidence intervals to determine where the null hypothesis has been rejected and where it has failed to be rejected).

For every 100 people treated with intensive treatment to below 120 mm Hg, there will be one more case of hypotension. It is important to be familiar with NNH. Especially when looking at SAE tables. They may not reflect mortality but SAEs that require hospitalization or additional medications introduce additional harms when you consider the primary outcomes of the clinical trial.

Table 3. Serious Adverse Events, Conditions of Interest, and Monitored Clinical Events.				
Variable	Intensive Treatment (N=4678)	Standard Treatment (N=4683)	Hazard Ratio	P Value
	no. of patients (%)			
Serious adverse event*	1793 (38.3)	1736 (37.1)	1.04	0.25
Conditions of interest				
Serious adverse event only				
Hypotension	110 (2.4)	66 (1.4)	1.67	0.001
Syncope	107 (2.3)	80 (1.7)	1.33	0.05
Bradycardia	87 (1.9)	73 (1.6)	1.19	0.28
Electrolyte abnormality	144 (3.1)	107 (2.3)	1.35	0.02
Injurious fall†	105 (2.2)	110 (2.3)	0.95	0.71
Acute kidney injury or acute renal failure‡	193 (4.1)	117 (2.5)	1.66	<0.001
Emergency department visit or serious adverse event				
Hypotension	158 (3.4)	93 (2.0)	1.70	<0.001
Syncope	163 (3.5)	113 (2.4)	1.44	0.003
Bradycardia	104 (2.2)	83 (1.8)	1.25	0.13
Electrolyte abnormality	177 (3.8)	129 (2.8)	1.38	0.006
Injurious fall†	334 (7.1)	332 (7.1)	1.00	0.97
Acute kidney injury or acute renal failure‡	204 (4.4)	120 (2.6)	1.71	<0.001
Monitored clinical events				
Adverse laboratory measure§				
Serum sodium <130 mmol/liter	180 (3.8)	100 (2.1)	1.76	<0.001
Serum sodium >150 mmol/liter	6 (0.1)	0		0.02
Serum potassium <3.0 mmol/liter	114 (2.4)	74 (1.6)	1.50	0.006
Serum potassium >5.5 mmol/liter	176 (3.8)	171 (3.7)	1.00	0.97
Orthostatic hypotension¶				
Alone	777 (16.6)	857 (18.3)	0.88	0.01
With dizziness	62 (1.3)	71 (1.5)	0.85	0.35

* A serious adverse event was defined as an event that was fatal or life-threatening, that resulted in clinically significant or persistent disability, that required or prolonged a hospitalization, or that was judged by the investigator to represent a clinically significant hazard or harm to the participant that might require medical or surgical intervention to prevent one of the other events listed above.
† An injurious fall was defined as a fall that resulted in evaluation in an emergency department or that resulted in hospitalization.
‡ Acute kidney injury or acute renal failure were coded if the diagnosis was listed in the hospital discharge summary and was believed by the safety officer to be one of the top three reasons for admission or continued hospitalization. A few cases of acute kidney injury were noted in an emergency department if the participant presented for one of the other conditions of interest.
§ Adverse laboratory measures were detected on routine or unscheduled tests; routine laboratory tests were performed at 1 month, then quarterly during the first year, then every 6 months.
¶ Orthostatic hypertension was defined as a drop in systolic blood pressure of at least 20 mm Hg or in diastolic blood pressure of at least 10 mm Hg at 1 minute after the participant stood up, as compared with the value obtained when the participant was seated. Standing blood pressures were measured at screening, baseline, 1 month, 6 months, 12 months, and yearly thereafter. Participants were asked if they felt dizzy at the time the orthostatic measure was taken.

I encourage you to dig into the data and see what you find. The press releases (in my opinion) gave quite a different impression prior to data release.

"This study provides potentially lifesaving information that will be useful to health care providers as they consider the best treatment options for some of their patients, particularly those over the age of 50," said Gary H. Gibbons, M.D., director of the National Heart, Lung, and Blood Institute (NHLBI), the primary sponsor of SPRINT. "We are delighted to have achieved this important milestone in the study in advance of the expected closure date for the SPRINT trial and look forward to quickly communicating the results to help inform patient care and the future development of evidence-based clinical guidelines."

This is a summary of the specific drug classes from the standard and intensive arms of the trial. I will let others debate the antihypertensive medication classes but it is noteworthy to observe how the data might have been influenced by variation in drug efficacy and safety in the populations studied.

Number of agents	Intensive (n=4678)	Standard (n=4683)
Average	2.7 (1.2)	1.8 (1.1)
0	125 (2.7)	530 (11.3)
1	493 (10.5)	1455 (31.1)
2	1429 (30.5)	1559 (33.3)
3	1486 (31.8)	807 (17.2)
4+	1137 (24.3)	323 (6.9)
ACE-I or angiotensin II antagonist	3580 (76.7)	2582 (55.2)
Renin inhibitors	1	1

Diuretics	3127 (67.0)	2006 (42.9)
Thiazide-type	2562 (54.9)	1557 (33.3)
Aldosterone receptor blockers	405 (8.7)	185 (4.0)
Other potassium-sparing diuretics	144 (3.1)	119 (2.5)
Alpha-1 blockers	482 (10.3)	258 (5.5)
Beta blockers	1919 (41.1)	1440 (30.8)
Central alpha-2 agonists or other centrally acting drugs	107 (2.3)	44 (0.9)
Calcium channel blockers	2667 (57.1)	1654 (35.4)
Direct vasodilators	340 (7.3)	110 (2.4)

A few notes:

There are challenges when looking at composite endpoints especially when time-to-event data may be impeded by a prior event. This clinical trial is reporting very different events at the 3.6-year mark then would be observed if the trial reported follow-up for the full 6 years.

The secondary outcomes included the individual measures of the composite outcome. As you can observe, several of the secondary measures failed to reject the null hypothesis. What happens if a patient's acute coronary syndrome is unobservable because the patient dies before the outcome is diagnosed? You can't assume that a subject will experience an event of interest if the follow-up period is shortened.

Framingham Risk Calculator vs. Reynolds Risk Score

It would be interesting to see clarification of selection of risk calculation tool. I am familiar with the debate about the estimated distributions of predicted risks in the population vary widely across models.

The Framingham Risk Calculator was the risk predictor tool for inclusion in the clinical trial and therefore influenced the baseline demographics of the clinical trial population.

Preventing Overdiagnosis

Benefits in clinical research are modeled as reduction in mortality, increase in life-years, survival rates, or quality adjusted life years.

Harms are modeled as increased rates in mortality, decrease in life-years or quality adjusted life years, or other surrogates (number of colonoscopies, number of false positives, biopsies, etc.)

The most important considerations when selecting an intervention at the point of care are the following:

- Do nothing (risk of no treatment vs. risk of intervention)
- Summarize harms for shared decision making
- Identify high-risk patients
- Provide a comparison of different treatment options

Complexity of screening algorithms

The debate surrounding risks associated with screening for disease upstream from actual illness has escalated with updated guidelines for breast and prostate cancer detection.

Improved skills in numeracy allow fully informed clinicians, patients, and journalists to carefully report the harms and benefits from randomized clinical trials and even observational trials with caution to only communicate reliable and accurate information.

When seeking to understand the vast literature it is helpful to identify the participant populations, interventions, and outcome measures. Different studies may capture all cause mortality, cancer mortality, only a specific type of cancer mortality, surgical interventions, presence of adjuvant therapy, and harms from screening.

Meta-analyses and systematic reviews often require careful attention to differences in randomization, populations, inclusion/exclusion criteria, follow-up, and if there may be outdated screening methodologies that would not be relevant or generizable to other datasets. For example, 5-year survival rate often is influenced by earlier detection—not necessarily meaningful improved outcomes such as mortality.

I suggest you read and review Screening for Breast Cancer with Mammography (Review) by the Cochrane Collaboration, Gotzsche PC, and Jorgensen KJ.

Trends in Metastatic Breast and Prostate Cancer — Lessons In Cancer Dynamics

H. Gilbert Welch M.D., M.P.H., David H. Gorski, M.D., Ph.D., and Peter C. Albertsen, M.D.

Conclusions

You survived the journey. The intention is that the travel guide helped navigate a bit of the "why" certain types of data are presented, what we can infer, and are those inferences valid. Although descriptive statistics simplifies concepts and provides a quick estimate of the central position of a frequency distribution or variation of a population they are only applicable to the data we have on hand. We can express measures of central tendency as parameters—they represent the whole population we are evaluating.

We discussed the limitations of sampling from the population. When we are evaluating samples we are using inferential statistics—not parameters—to make generalizations about the larger population from which the samples were drawn. The caution is that you are providing data about a population that you have not fully measured, and therefore, cannot ever be completely sure that the values/statistics you calculate are correct. The majority of inferential tests require you to make informed and theory based guesses to understand or design the inferential tests—I hope you arrive safely—and confidently.

Statistics are no substitute for judgment--

Henry Clay

More information on literacy

The National Academies of Sciences, Engineering, and Medicine.

2015. Health literacy: Past, present,

and future: Workshop summary. Washington,

DC: The National Academies Press.

IOM (Institute of Medicine). 2014. Health Literacy and Numeracy: Workshop Summary. Washington, DC: The National Academies Press.

U.S. Department of Health and Human Services, Office of Disease Prevention and Health Promotion. (2010). National Action Plan to Improve Health Literacy. Washington, DC

DeWalt DA, Callahan LF, Hawk VH, Broucksou KA, Hink A, Rudd R, Brach C. Health Literacy Universal Precautions Toolkit. (Prepared by North Carolina Network Consortium, The Cecil G. Sheps Center for Health Services Research, The University of North Carolina at Chapel Hill, under Contract No. HHSA290200710014.) AHRQ Publication No. 10-0046-EF) Rockville, MD. Agency for Healthcare Research and Quality. April 2010.

Important Websites to follow:

Meta-Research Innovation Center at Stanford (METRICS) http://metrics.stanford.edu

STATS http://www.stats.org

Medicine in Media

http://www.vaoutcomes.org/resources/resourcesandtips/primers/

TheBMJ http://www.bmj.com/us/news/analysis

Care that mattershttp://www.carethatmatters.org/info/

Choosing Wisely http://www.choosingwisely.org

Health News Reviewhttp://www.healthnewsreview.org

National Physician Alliance http://www.npalliance.org

Lown Conference http://lowninstitute.org

Preventing Overdiagnosis http://www.preventingoverdiagnosis.net

###

Thank you for joining me on this data journey. If you enjoyed it, won't you please take a moment to leave me a review at your favorite retailer?

Thanks!

Bonny

Connect with me:

Twitter: http://twitter.com/graphemeconsult or http://twitter.com/dataanddonuts

Subscribe to my blog: http://www.dataanddonuts.org

http://alzheimersdiseasethebrand.com